Hair Growth Genie

W FOSTER

ISBN: 1461183596
ISBN-13: 9781461183594

DEDICATION

To all women (and men) who strive to have long, healthy hair. May your journey be filled with success and always enjoy the ride.

CONTENTS

ACKNOWLEDGMENTS

My family for enduring my endless hair growth experiments.
The following hair growth forums for their endless list of experiments and tips:
www.longhaircareforum.com
www.blackhaircare.com

ABOUT THE HAIR GROWTH GENIE

The average person has over 100 000 hairs on their head. Hair grows on average less than half an inch a month (1.25 cm), that's on average 6 inches a year. To attain long hair you would have to wait between 3-5 years! That is provided you lose none of your hair, your ends do not break off and you maintain average growth with no cutting!

After years of personal research on hair growth, I finally found all the things in combination that allows anyone to achieve optimal healthy hair growth of up to double the normal growth, that is up to 3/4 inches per month or more.

Many might doubt whether this is in fact true - I can guarantee you it is. Not only this, but using the secrets from this book, my hair was transformed from bleached dry, slow growing hair to a healthy and growing hair.

I wrote the Hair Growth Genie as a bible of tips and tricks as well as daily and weekly regimes for all hair types. Women with straight, wavy, curly, thick, thin any hair can achieve beautiful and luscious hair growth by following the Hair Growth Genie guide.

I've also included a free Hair Regime Journal, which you can print out, and use to track your growth.

Good luck on your journey, may it be a long, beautiful and abundantly satisfying one!

The Truth About Hair Growth

Before you embark on your hair growth journey, it is important to understand hair growth. Why do some people seem blessed with fast hair growth and healthy hair - even people with the same type of hair as you and you don't?

Well here's the not so secret secret - your hair is growing. Don't believe me? Have you ever noticed that you dye your hair - a few weeks or months later you see a ton of regrowth - but your actual hair length does not seem to have changed/grown. Or you relax your hair, and you know your hair is growing because you can tell from the regrowth. Your hair has grown - you have just not done enough to maintain the growth. You've lost the length you grew due to breakage or shedding. Some people think that their hair shrinks, it does not shrink, and it is breaking off at the ends.

The reality is that even though everyone's hair grows - it's about keeping the length that does grow, not just about growing it. Many don't eat the right foods or receive sufficient nutrients to encourage growth and maintain healthy hair, they don't use the right products to optimally grow hair and most importantly, they don't maintain their hair once it does grow.

If you analyzed your hair - you would find those tiny white dots on the ends - that is where hair has broken off. You might find that your ends are dry, crunchy, straggly or thinner than at the root - this is where split ends have split and broken off leaving a thin trail.

You might find that you wake up with a mass of knots; this is where your split ends are creating friction and tangling and damaging the healthy hairs.

When you rip the brush through your wet hair - you are not aware of all the hairs you are ripping apart - resulting in broken off hair, split ends and damage to previously healthy hair.

If you have bleached your hair - whether it's a full head, highlights or lowlights, you have effectively decreased the volume of each hair that was bleached and made it five times more vulnerable to breakage, splitting and sheer damage.

Hair Growth Phases

Hair growth is divided into three different cycles of growth or phases. They are known as the Anagen. Catagen and Telogen phase.

Anagen is the growth phase. Catagen is the regressing phase. Telogen is the resting phase. Each phase also has an Exogen sub-phase, which is an exiting phase that is when hair tends to shed - when it's reached the end of its cycle. Shedding is normal, and happens with any human being. We shed on average 100 hairs a day. If your hair is straight you won't really notice it, however if your hair is curly you'll notice the hairs when you touch your hair as they have been caught in the curls and come loose as you manipulate your hair. It's not that you are losing more hair than before -but rather it's more obvious than if your hair was straightened and it shed throughout the day on its own.

Normally 90% of hair is in the Anagen phase at any given time, while 10-14% are in the Telogen phase and 1-2% n the Catagen phase. This is good news as it means that most of your hair is growing most of the time!

The growth phase for hair on the head lasts 2-7 years. At the end of the Anagen phase, a signal causes the hair to go into the Catagen (regressing) phrase. During this phase, the hair growth stops for 2-3 weeks while a club hair is formed ending just prior to the Telogen (resting) phase kicking in.

During the Telogen (resting) phase, the club hair, which began forming in the Catagen stages, is now fully formed. It is now a dead fully keratinized hair. Hair is normally shed at this phase as well. We can of course minimize the abnormal hair shedding/breakage that is not due to the Telogen phase.

The length of the Anagen (growing) phase is genetically pre-determined. We thus cannot change how long our hair grows for and stays on our head - what we can however change - is how we treat the hair that does come out to make it last as long as the Anagen/Catagen/Telogen phase allows it.

This means that every person is on average capable of keeping up to an average of 3 years growth on our heads which is normally 18-24 inches of hair length.

These are all average statistics. Now imagine if you went above the average by treating your hair above the average?

Hair Like Silk

Before we continue on the Hair Growth journey, I would like to share this little story with you.

Each time you are tempted to mistreat your hair, I would like you to remember the phrase "Hair Like Silk" and this is why:

Hair can be likened to a piece of silk. Can you imagine been given a delicate piece of beautiful black silk and being asked to take care of it for three years.

Each day you look at the piece of silk and each day you are reminded how beautiful it is. You love to touch it, twirl the silk in your hands, and feel it on your skin. The beautiful silk gives you immense joy as it's longevity depends on you, the quality depends on you - and it's your responsibility to ensure that piece of silk remains as beautiful as it was the day you received it.

Now imagine washing that piece of silk with a harsh detergent. You then put your blow dryer on its highest heat setting in order to dry it. You follow that through with ripping a brush onto the piece of silk. You then flat iron the silk until it's shiny and smooth. All you've done is smooth down the rough edges, which will reappear once you wash it again. You then throw some bleach onto the silk. Hating the color, you dye it back to its original color. You then throw it into the swimming pool without any covering and go through the routine again.

You get my drift don't you? So remember "Hair Like Silk".

Hair Damage Reality Check

Deciding to embark on a healthy hair growth journey is great - however you need to keep reminding yourself why you are doing it. Long hair is wonderful and is a by-product of treating your hair like silk. There will always be temptations to bleach your hair or dye it or iron it, just remember that all of these chemically or mechanically damage your hair and will set your hair growth back as you will need to do that much more to get it back to health so it can continue to grow.

Below are pictures of damaged and healthy hair under a microscope. So think carefully, perhaps use this page as a reference every time you are tempted to alter the natural state of your hair. Ultimately your natural state is the best - and you can only see it once you get your hair back to optimal health.

Setting A Hair Growth Goal

Determine Your Hair Growth Goal

Before you decide to do anything in life, including growing your hair, it's important to set a goal.

The most common way to measure hair growth goals is by setting measurable targets according to your body. The targets are set by a visual cue that you can use to visually check on your growth and goal.

Hair is measured from the centre of the hair line (where your hair starts above your nose) to the longest point at the back of your head. Hair length and the various hair length goals can be set as follows:

- Bald - having no hair at all on the head
- Shaved - hair that is completely shaved down to the scalp
- Stubble- very short hairs that doesn't cover the skin completely
- Buzz - hair that is extremely short and hardly there
- Cropped- hair that is a little longer than a buzz
- Boy Cut- hair that is longer than a crop, but not yet hits the ears
- Ear length - hair up to one's ears
- Chin level - hair grows down to the chin
- Flip level - hair reaching the neck or shoulders
- Shoulder length - hair reaching the shoulders

- Armpit Length - hair that reaches the armpit
- Bra Strap level - this is where your hair reaches your bra strap, in between armpit and mid back length
- Mid back level - hair that's at about the same point as the widest part of one's ribcage and chest area
- Waist length - hair that falls at the smallest part of one's waist, a little bit above the hip bones
- Tailbone length - hair that is at about the area of one's tailbone
- Classic length - hair that reaches where one's legs meet his or her buttocks
- Thigh length - hair that is at the mid-thigh
- Knee-length - hair that is at the knee
- Calf length - hair that is at the calf
- Floor length - hair that reaches the floor

Setting hair growth goals would be based on the next point. E.g. if your hair is currently Arm Pit Length, the next goal would Bra Strap Length.

Because hair grows on average 1/2 inch per month - your goal would be to increase this growth to 1 inch per month using the techniques in this book. Thus you would measure from your armpit to your bra strap, how many inches growth it would be - thus you would know how many months until your goal could be reached.

An example of setting a hair growth goal would be as follows:

Current hair length: Arm Pit Length (APL)
Goal length: Bra Strap Length (BSL)
Inches to goal: 4 inches
Months to goal: 4 months
Current Month: August
Goal month: December

Thus your goal would be:
I intend to grow my hair from APL to BSL by December 2010. I will do this through following my hair growth regime. Once you have reached your goal you would then set your next goal.

Reaching Your Goal

Reaching your hair growth goal will take a lot of discipline. You will need to stay focused. As with any goal, it is important to visualize the end result.

Some tips to visualizing your hair growth goal:
Cut out some photos of your goal length
Start a hair growth journal where you can write down your goal and paste the photos of your goal (Your free printable journal included see back of the book)
Print out the hair care regime guide at the back of the book
Read the daily affirmation
Daily Affirmation For Hair Growth

It goes without saying that you have to believe in anything that you set out to do. This affirmation should be said daily to motivate you on your hair growth journey. Say it when you are combing your hair at night or after writing in your journal whilst picturing yourself getting compliments on your hair growth when it reaches your goal length.

Take a deep breath and feel your scalp becoming relaxed. Visualize the hairs having an open field in which to grow abundantly. Say:

"I bless my hair with love. I am grateful for my hair continuing to grow long, healthy, abundantly and strong.

Before You Cut Your Hair

Many people will tell you that you have to trim your hair every 6 weeks to encourage growth. This is a myth. Your hair will grow regardless of whether you cut it or not. The key to growing your hair longer is to maintain the old hair and encourage new growth.

If you have damaged ends, most likely the damage extends quite far up the hair shaft. The truth is that the damage will most likely travel further up and cause your hair condition to look terrible and crunchy. For most this would mean one major chop. If you are comfortable with starting fresh, then of course go for it, your hair growth journey will just be made longer.

However, you can get around this. By doing micro trims which are smaller trims done over a period of time rather than one big chop. Essentially you trim only 1/8" (less than a cm) every few weeks. Your hair will continue to grow - and you would be slowly cutting off the damage. Because you would also be maintaining you hair - you are acting to prevent further damage and keep the current damage under control.

You can both go to a hairdresser and discuss this plan with her so she understands. You might be met with many that will tell you this is not true - but be strong. It's your hair!

One of the biggest secrets to growing long hair besides maintaining growth - is simply not cutting. You only need micro trims to cut off only the damaged hair and not the healthy hairs. This is a longer method, but worthwhile in the long run.

You can also do it yourself. You have to purchase a high quality small hair scissors with very sharp blades. You would section your hair off into thin parts. Sit under a bright light in front of a close up mirror. If you hair is longer than should length, you can wear a black top, as the split ends show better on a dark background.

Else cut the ends only in the daytime in a brightly lit area for maximum visibility of split ends. Cut only the split ends from each section. Don't touch the hair that does not have split ends. If you see a white dot on your hair shaft - this is the point where you hair is going to break off and causes tangles - cut slightly above the white dot.

Tie the pieces that are done and put it aside so that you do not cut the same sections.

Once you are done, rub Jojoba oil any other oil or serum that you are comfortable with onto your ends to maintain them and keep them moisturized. The ends are the oldest on your entire head and need a lot of moisture as natural oils from your scalp to not get to the ends easily. Oil your ends daily to keep them moisturized.

What is Your Hair Type

Before we go into diagnosing problems with your hair and following a hair regime, you need to understand what your hair type is and how porous it is. Hair types are there as a visual aid and in conjunction with texture and porosity (your hairs ability to retain moisture or product) assists with which products and regimes work best for you.

Did you know there are 11 hair sub-types of hair? These sub-types fall into 4 main hair types, which are Types 1, 2, 3 and 4. Within these main types, there are sub categories that determine the texture of your hair. It is important to recognize what your hair type is so that you will know which methods/routines would work best for or against you. This doesn't change the standard hair routine that should be followed, but will affect how you treat your hair and what products you use.

Type 1 - Straight

1a - stick straight
1b - straight but with a slight body wave, just enough to add some volume, doesn't look wavy
1c - straight with body wave and one or two visible S-waves (e.g. nape of neck or temples)

Type 2 - Wavy

2a - loose, stretched out S-waves throughout the hair. Very fine, thin and fairly easy to handle. Is easily straightened or curled.

2b - shorter, more distinct S-waves (similar to waves from braiding damp hair). Medium textures and resistant to styling, has a tendency to frizz.

2c - distinct S-waves and the odd spiral curl forming here and there. Normally thick and course textured and resistant to styling and frizzes easily.

Type 3 - Curly

3a - big, loose spiral curls, usually shiny

3b - bouncy ringlets, medium curl to loose corkscrews

3c - Tight corkscrews, kinky, tightly curled with lots of strands packed together.

Type 4 - Curly / Kinky

4a - tightly coiled S-curls when stretched

4b - tightly coiled hair bending in Z angles, prone to shrinking up to 75% of actual hair length.

Porosity

Porosity is the hairs ability to absorb moisture. So the more porous your hair, the more open your cuticles are which means it's easier and quicker to get color or product into the hair shaft. The cuticle is the overlapping hair scale on the hair shaft. However it also means that moisture leaves your hair just as quickly. You are thus prone to dry, brittle looking hair. If your hair is not that porous, it means your cuticles lie flatter, your hair retains its moisture for longer, and generally your hair is healthier. Only proper care over a period of time will slowly close the cuticle and make your hair less porous.

Low Porosity = Flat cuticles, difficult to get moisture, product or color into hair

Normal Porosity = Slightly raised cuticle, retains moisture, harder to get product and color into hair

High Porosity = Very raised cuticles, loses moisture quickly, easy to get product and color into hair

High porosity hair is the most prone to damage and dryness. The best thing for high porous hair is Apple Cider Vinegar rinses (recipe further on), which closes the cuticle thus locking in hairs moisture.

To determine whether your hair is low or high porosity - feel it. If it feels dry and crunchy when dry and rubbery when wet it is probably due to high porosity and will benefit from deep treatments and Apple Cider Vinegar rinses as well as acid (pH) balancing conditioners.

Hair care products to avoid

Before we get to Hair Growth and Care regimes, it's important to understand the products you use on your hair, which ones to avoid and which ones are best, as well as dispelling some hair myths. There is no point putting products on your hair, if you don't understand what it's doing now, and what it's doing in the long run.

The Hair care industry is worth billions of dollars each year. There are of course products that are excellent in assisting with the condition of the hair and a lot of research has been put into these products. However there are also many products whose ingredients only mask the underlying damage and do nothing to actually treat the symptoms.

You might look at it and think that if it's making your hair look good then you don't care - but understand that products that mask damage and cause more damage, leads to your hair breaking and splitting. So it might look good now, but ultimately you will be losing that lovely length you are trying so hard to retain.

Regardless of the texture of your hair -there are ingredients in products that are either carcinogens (poisons) or cause more damage to your hair than good over the long run.

Did you know that 100 years ago the rate of cancer was 1 out of every 100 people in the USA and in 2010 it is currently 1 in every 3?

There are many contributors to cancer: pollution, air quality, water quality, food quality, noise pollution, technological pollution (think of all the wireless beams in the air) and lack of sufficient nutrients in our mostly modified food.

The reality is that we as consumers don't receive full disclosure from the manufacturers of beauty products, because quite frankly why would they want to warn us when they don't have to. Because the beauty industry is not classified as medical - full disclosure is not a legal requirement in most countries in the world. You might see warnings on household detergents but that is the extent of it.

As consumers we should educate ourselves on what we are consuming internally and externally. The little we know can go along way not just to great hair, but great health as well.

So lets go. This list is only a list of the most common ones - there are however thousands out there. If you would like to see a full list then please see the links in the Resources section at the end of the book.

If you see any of these ingredients, then by all means avoid in any beauty products, hair, skin or body:

Hair Spray

Scientists conducted a study in the UK and found that women who use hairspray containing an ingredient called phthalates during the first trimester of pregnancy increased the chances of having a son with a genetic deformity in the urinary tract. They found that taking folic acid supplements decreased the risk, but that does not mean it eliminates it. They also found an increased risk in women who worked in industries where they are exposed to hairspray chemicals such as hair product factories, research laboratories and hair salons.

Propylene Glycol

Propylene Glycol is a common humectants (attracts moisture) in cosmetics. It is also the major ingredient in anti freeze products, brake fluid and hydraulic fluid. Tests found that it is a skin irritant and research warns that you should avoid skin contact and can cause liver abnormalities and kidney failure. Exposure through inhalation causes nausea, vomiting and central nervous system depression.

Mineral Oil/Petrolatum/Petroleum/Coal Tar

Mineral Oil, Petrolatum, Petroleum and Coal Tar are all derived from crude oil. These ingredients are used as a metal cutting fluid. Research has found that this liquid suffocates the skin by forming an oil film. So your hair and skin looks shiny, but in reality oxygen and moisture is being blocked out. Holding large amounts of moisture in the hair and skin can also result in long-term immature, unhealthy and sensitive skin that dries out easily. This results in premature aging.

Sodium Lauryl Sulfate (SLS) and Sodium Laureth Sulfate

This is a common one found in MOST shampoos. There are however a number that do not contain these ingredients. SLS is a skin irritant and used in order to test the healing properties of other ingredients. So they use SLS to cause a skin irritation in order to test a product that will ease the irritation! SLS also dries out the hair due to its detergent effect. SLS is also used more commonly in household detergents, garage floor cleaners, engine degreasers and car wash soaps.

Sulfates have been found to cause poisonous nitrates and dioxins to form in shampoo and cleansers by reacting with commonly used ingredients found in many other products. Large amounts of nitrates can enter the body from just one shampoo application.

A derivative called "Sodium Fluoride" is used in certain brands of toothpaste and also as a rat poison! In order to counteract the effects of SLS on hair, laboratories developed conditioners. The conditioners re-close the open cuticle from the harsh sulfates and using ingredients based on silicone, the damage is masked by creating a waterproof seal on the hair. The problem is that this seal also blocks out moisture and hides the damage.

Silicone

Silicone based conditioners and hair products contain ingredients typically ending in the words "cone", "conol" or "xane". In no way is damage eliminated, but rather hidden by the cones. How do you treat damage that you can't see? The damage is still there leading to more damage, which leads to breakage and dryness of your hair, which results in a longer struggle to grow your hair and get it to its optimal healthy state.

Many conditioners do not contain cones and are generally healthier for hair. When you first cut cones out of your conditioners or leave INS, your hair will seem more damaged, this is because the damage is no longer hidden. As you begin to treat your hair and follow a hair care regime, slowly this damage will be healed and you can move on cone free!

Glycerin (synthetic)

Glycerin draws moisture from inside the skin or hair, and holds it on the surface for a better "feel". Because it's drawing moisture from inside the skin and hair, once the Glycerin is off, the hair and skin are left bone dry. Glycerin is listed as a hazardous collagen.

Elastin

Elastin comes from animal skins and ground up chicken feet. It creates a film that suffocates and over moisturizes the skin. Many soap bars are made from lye and animal fat. The animal fat has the potential to allow bacteria to feed and grow in it. It also results in the corrosion and drying out of skin.

Derivatives are found in most cosmetic crème such as pro collagen, collagen, hyaluronic acid etc, all of which cannot penetrate the skin due to the high molecular weight, so they act as a coat and nothing else.

Other useless ingredients are insoluble oil-based Vitamin A (Retinal Palmitate), Placental Extracts, and Royal Bee Jelly (more on that soon).

Biotin (external)

Biotin is a wonderful supplement to take internally to promote hair growth. A deficiency of this supplement has been associated with greasy scalps, hair loss and balding. It is however very rare in humans. It is a good idea to take it as a supplement, but there is no need to take large doses, as it is unnecessary.

External products that contain Biotin are however quite simply a myth. The molecular structure of Biotin is too large to penetrate the skin or hair and thus is used more for marketing that any benefit.

Lanolin

Lanolin is a common skin sensitizer, which can cause allergic skin rashes. It contains pesticides and dioxins used on sheep and wool.

Lauramide

Lauramide is often used in cosmetic products to thicken and allow the product to lather. It is most often in creams, shampoos and soap liquids. It is also used in dishwashing detergents for its grease cutting abilities. It is extremely drying to hair and can cause skin and scalp irritation such as itching and allergic reactions. Lauramide has been declared a carcinogen.

Hair Product Lies

Now that you know what's in those products you are using - lets take a look at marketing myths used to sell more hair and skin products.

Natural Products - Are They Really Natural?

In cosmetic, food and product terminology, the term "natural" is used when the manufacturer does not use more than 70% organic ingredients and methods and thus would not get a government certification to certify the products as organic.

Thus the only word that matters are "Organic" and not "Natural" The manufacturers know this. They have to comply with a ton of standards in order to simply get their products on the shelves. They however also know that it is a lot more expensive to make organic products, as organic farming is a small percentage compared to the majority.

Organic means that products or food are made avoiding any synthetic chemicals and the farm is free of synthetic chemicals used in irrigation. The level to determine the labeling of natural or organic products is as follows. Look at the labels to give you an idea of just how many ingredients are indeed organic.

Labels as follows:
"100% Organic" -products made with entirely certified organic materials and methods

"Organic" - products made with 95% organic materials and methods

"Made with organic ingredients" - products made with 70% organic materials and methods

"Natural" - used by manufacturers who have failed to meet the standards to be certified as "organic"

The only exception to "Natural" products are if the product has a Natural Products Association (NPA) certification that certifies that the product uses 95% truly natural ingredients excluding water (e.g. Plant and mineral based) with no toxins harmful to humans.

The NPA warns consumers to look out for the following top ten marketing foolery on products:

- Made with organic essential oils
- Contains organic ingredients
- Made with nontoxic ingredients
- 100 percent natural
- Essentially nontoxic
- Earth-friendly
- Environmentally safer
- Hypoallergenic/Dermatologist Tested/Allergy Tested/Non-Irritating
- Vegan
- Cruelty-Free

They also warn that the US Food & Drug Administration only certifies food products as organic. This means that plant based products or ingredients are not certified by the FDA at all so may include harmful by products or have been farmed with chemical fertilizers, toxic pesticides and other harsh chemicals.

The wonderful thing about home made recipes for hair care is that a lot of them are food based, so if you want to go all the way, then buy 100% organic honey, avocados, dairy etc to use in your hair care recipes.

PH Levels

PH stands for the power of the hydrogen atom. Skin and hair are said to have a pH of 5.0. A scale from 0 to 14 is used to measure acidity and alkalinity of solutions. PH 7.0 is neutral.

There is no such thing as a "pH balanced" product because a product's pH will drift during shelf life and alter when applied to the hair and skin.

A product's pH is not a danger to the body, but the synthetic chemicals used in cosmetics – often to alter the pH to please the ones who fall for the "pH balanced" story – are.

In a nutshell...

Thus you can see that you should never simply trust the marketing or labels - no matter how natural or organic they say the product is - the best judge is to check the labeling for wording and certifications and read the ingredients list. Armed with the basics as above, you can now try to avoid the carcinogens that could damage your health in the long term. Your best options are to look at products that are as organic as possible, or make them yourself from raw ingredients.

Your Hair Regime

Remember your hair is always growing and the tips will speed it up you have to however retain the hair to see it. To do this you have to follow a hair regime.

Regardless of whether your hair is oily or dry, following a regime will slowly get rid of the conditions that cause your hair to be excessively oily or dry and normalize it to a healthy state.

You might read the list of oils and conditioners and wonder how it will help an oily scalp. Oil is overly produced when the scalp is dry from the harsh shampoos used. Once your regime is in swing, your scalp will return to a healthy state and will not need to over produce oil.

Weekly Regime

The following regime should be followed as closely as possible to achieve optimal results. It can be used on any hair type of any length.

1. Pre-oil your dry unwashed hair by massaging any mixture of hair oils (see recipes or use pure coconut oil) into the scalp, lengths and ends of your hair. The easiest way to do this is to part your into four sections. Rub

the oil between your palms to heat it. Massage into the hair until your hair is saturated with oil.

2. Cover with a wrap, shower cap or hot towels for 30 minutes. If you are using hot towel, you will need to reheat the towel under hot water once it cools down. You may also sit under a dryer or heat cap for 15 minutes.

3. Wash your hair with a gentle sulfate free shampoo if you are using shampoo or a light cheap conditioner if you are using conditioner only wash (read more about this later).

Afterwards, apply a Moisturizing Conditioner/Treatment (see recipes for home made options)

Comb through with a wide toothcomb or your fingers and rinse thoroughly Gently dab excess water out of your hair with paper towel or a micro fiber towel. Do not use a terry cloth towel on your hair as it causes frizz.

Apply a leave in conditioner or light serum o light oil such as Jojoba on your ends. You may also use a drop of honey mixed into your leave in if you plan to air dry.

Style your hair.

Daily Regime

The daily regime should be followed every single day whether it's washday or not.

1. Take specific vitamins for hair growth daily
2. Cover hair with a satin bonnet, satin scarf or sleep on a silk/satin pillowcase
3. Drink 8 glasses of water
4. Try to do some form of exercise for a minimum of 15 minutes or tilt your head for 5 minutes
5. Massage your head without oil for 5 minutes daily (Read the section o Head Massage for more details)
6. Apply a serum, jojoba or coconut oil to the ends daily

Washing Your Hair

Washing your every day can strip the hair of natural oils and also cause further damage by over exposure to harsh sulfates, sodium chloride (salt) and other chemicals present in most store bought shampoos. The optimal wash period should be no more than twice a week depending on your schedule.

E.g. Monday and Thursdays would be your washdays.

Shampoo once only. There are different methods of washing hair - however washing only once with sulfate free shampoo or conditioner wash (without shampoo) is the best options.

Shampoos containing the ingredient "Sulfate" should be avoided as they strip the hair. Examples include "Ammonium Laureth Sulfate", "Ammonium Lauryl Sulfate","Tea Laureth Sulphate", "Tea Lauryl Sulfate" or "Sodium Lauryl Sulfate". The only sulfates that are considered gentle are:
- Sodium Myreth Sulphate
- Polyoxethylene Fatty Alcohols
- PEG 80
- Sorbitan Laurate
- Decyl Polyglucose
- Cocamidopropyl Betaine
- Sodium Myreth Sulfate

Clarifying shampoos like Pantenes should not be used more than once a month. These will contain sulfates used to remove product build.

If you are doing a conditioner only wash, then you might want to do a once a month clean with shampoo, but rather opt for a sulfate free version.

Ensure that you don't pile hair on top of your hair when washing. Leave it to hang down to prevent matting or tangling. Put shampoo on your fingertips and wash your scalp. There is no need to scrub the hair - as the lengths and ends will be washed from the run down of water and suds from your scalp.

Washing hair is important to get rid of dirt and grime that may block hair follicles, thus not allowing the hair follicles enough oxygen for optimal growth.

If you are doing a conditioner wash and your hair does not "feel" clean - then ensure that you use a lot of conditioner and allow it to sit on your head for at least 5 minutes while you massage your scalp and hair with your fingertips.

Before You Wash

One day before or an hour before is the best time to infuse your hair with additional moisture it needs for optimal growth. This period can be used to apply hot oil treatments, which will be washed out from the shampoo.

Ideal hot oil treatments need not be expensive purchases. There are recipes in the book for inexpensive oil treatments that you can use. Coconut oil is the best oil to be used for the mid lengths and ends of hair as it have the highest absorption rate (i.e. it penetrates the hair better than any other oils). Most other oils only coat the hair shaft. Olive oil can also be used but if you can go for Extra Virgin Olive Oil.

Rosemary Essential Oil can also be added (a few drops) which stimulates the scalp. Indian hair oils such as Amla, Bhinjri etc can also be used.

It should always be heated for approximately 10 seconds in a microwave or over a bowl of boiling water.

Oil should be massaged into the lengths, ends and scalp for a minimum of 5 minutes. The hair should then be covered with a damp hot towel or plastic cap for 30 minutes. You can also sit under a hood hair dryer or manual dryer for 15 minutes if you don't have enough time.

Shampooing

Once your pre-washing oiling is completed, you would then need to wash the oils out with Shampoo or Conditioner.

Other "Shampoo" Methods

Traditionally we wash our hair with shampoo, rinse and then condition. However much research and trials have been carried out by various women as a result there are other Shampoo methods. The best thing to do to find the right one for you is to alternative by trying different ones. If you do decide to try a different "shampoo" method - it will only be worth it to try it for at least 4 weeks to allow your hair to get used to the method and settle.

Alternative Shampoo Method:

CO - Conditioner or condition-only washing method - this method is recommended for those with thick, curly, dry or frizz prone hair. Any conditioner is used the same as a shampoo on the hair and scalp. With this method however you have to spend more time really massaging the conditioner gently into the hair and scalp for longer than you normally would with shampoo. Many report softer, frizz free hair. If you have fine hair, then this method is not recommended.

CWC - You first Condition the hair with Conditioner, followed by a wash with a sulfate free shampoo, followed by a conditioner.

WCWC - Various hair salons use this method and they swear by the conditioning properties. It is simply a Wash; Condition with a Protein based conditioner, Wash, and then Condition with moisture rich conditioner.

WO - Water only washing method. This method is used by a lot of women who do not want to use shampoo or conditioner on their hair. Hair is washed with water only and rinsed thoroughly, followed by hair oils for moisture sealing.
This method relies on the oils and hairs natural oils to moisturize the hair.

Shampoo Bars - A Shampoo Bar is a soap bar made with a mixture of oil and lye. It contains a lot less harsh chemicals than shampoo. The pH level however interferes with the natural acidity of the skin and therefore an Apple Cider Vinegar rinse is always done after using a shampoo bar.

Herbs - Many people use a mixture of Indian herbs such as Neem, Shikakai, Brahmi and normal Catnip as a shampoo on their hair. The herbs are infused into water, filtered and used as a shampoo rinse.

Protein Treatments

Hair conditioning has to maintain a balance between protein and moisture in order to grow. Most chemical processes such as perms, bleaching, relaxers, colors, bleaching etc strip protein from the hair. It is thus essential to have a protein treatment following any chemical treatment.
Protein treatments are to be followed by a moisturizing treatment to maintain the balance and condition of the hair. For severely damaged hair they can be done once a week initially - and then every second week once your hair health has improved.

Once your hair becomes healthy, this can be cut to once a month.

Protein treatments can either be leave in or rinse out. They should always be applied to towel dried clean hair with no conditioner.

Treatments should be combed through and left on the hair for 30-60 minutes before rinsing (or left in if using a leave in treatment).

A moisturizing conditioner should always follow protein treatments. It should state "Moisturizing" on the bottle; else use one of the home made moisturizing treatments.

With a leave in Protein treatment it would be left in the hair after conditioning.

Moisture Treatments

Daily wear; Blow-drying, ironing or applying any heat to your hair removes moisture. You would thus need to replace lost moisture with every wash.

Moisturizing treatments or Conditioners should be applied after every wash and after every protein treatment.

Deep conditioning with specific deep moisture treatments should be done weekly on your hair washdays.

For best results it should be left in for 20-60 minutes with heat.

Hair Diagnosis

The routine in this book works on all hair types - however you may experience problems with your hair that does not seem to go away no matter what you do and it seems to get worse.

Below is a quick diagnosis of the symptoms and solutions to try. It's important to follow through a process of elimination.

Problem: Hair is suddenly tangling easily; looks dull and frazzled, ends are crunchy and dry, hair feel straw like

Pre-Diagnosis: Your hair could have product build up. To test these do the following:

Your hair needs to be clarified (cleansing on steroids if you will!) first to remove all product residues on your hair. You will need a Clarifying shampoo such as Pantene Clarifying, Suave, Neutrogena or VO5 Kiwi Lime Shampoo. They unfortunately contain Sulfates, but will work to quickly remove buildup. Wash your hair twice with the clarifying shampoo. This is the only time you should ever wash your hair twice. Do not condition your hair after this. Leave your hair to air dry on it's own.

Alternatively you can follow up a normal non-Sulfate shampoo wash, also twice, with Apple Vinegar rinse using a 1/2-cup of Apple

Cider Vinegar to a jug of water. Again leaving your hair to dry on it's own.

Your hair will feel extremely "tight" and squeaky, however this is temporary to allow you to diagnose the problem.
Next step is to feel your hair.

Diagnosis #1: Too Much Protein
If your hair feels crunchy, bunching up, dry or brittle - chances are that you have too much protein in your hair and need a moisturizing treatment.

Solution: Apply a deep moisturizing conditioner or treatment of your choice into your hair. Wrap with a shower cap or towel and sit under a hooded dryer for 15 minutes or heated towels for 30-60 minutes. You may leave it on longer if you choose

Diagnosis #2: **Too Little Protein**
If your hair feels thin, transparent, and wiry and the ends seem see through, with rough feel to the strands, then you need protein in your hair.

Solution: You need to apply a deep protein treatment to your hair of your choice, followed by a moisturizing treatment to add moisture back into the hair as protein hardens the hair.

Diagnosis #3: Need Moisture
If your hair feels fine but is lacking body then you need moisture

Solution: Apply a moisture treatment as above.

If your hair is a combination of the above, then try one thing at a time, but always include the moisture treatment. The Emergency Treatment in this book is a great moisture treatment to use on hair that needs a boost.

Styling Your Hair

With heat

When you are trying to grow your hair, it is advisable to use heat as sparingly as possible. If you have to heat style your hair, then rather air dry first.

The best way to air dry hair if you plan to style it with heat, is to comb your hair around your head, this is called wrapping, and then putting a stocking or cling wrap over your hair. Allow to air dry to as dry as possible before using heat.

Some people's hair unfortunately cannot straighten from low or no heat settings, so if you must use heat, wait until your hair is as naturally dried as possible to minimize the amount of heat used on the hair.

Using curling or hot irons is never recommended. However if you must use a styling iron, do so only once a week and only on dry hair with a heat protection serum. Do not use styling irons if you have hair oil or silicone on your hair. You are literally frying your hair. The silicone will mask the damage until your next wash.

The best time to style your hair with heat, is after a moisturizing treatment when your hair is amply protected.

Without heat for curly or wavy hair

No heat is always the best option if you can get away with it. Some options to style your hair with no heat are the following:

- Plopping - for curly or wavy textures
- Apply a leave in conditioner, hair serum or light hair oil such as Coconut, Jojoba, Olive oil or Almond oil to your hair. You can also mix in a drop of pure honey for additional softness and shine.
- Comb through with a wide toothcomb or preferably your fingers.
- Spread an old t-shirt or micro-fiber towel onto a flat surface (such as the toilet with seat down).
- Bend over at the waist and position your hair in the middle of the cloth.
- Pile your hair to the top of your hair.
- With your head touching the cloth, drape the back section of cloth over your head.
- Twist the sides until they form "sausage rolls" and clip or tie them at the base of your neck.
- After 15-30 minutes remove the cloth. If your hair is frizzy after plopping lightly graze the hair with gel.
- Then remove the T shirt and shake your head gently
- Your hair will now have beautiful waves or curls depending on the texture of your hair
- After this - do not touch your hair at all. Any hair manipulation will cause your hair to frizz

Bunning or braiding - for any hair texture

Bunning is an easy style where you tie your hair up into a low or high ponytail, and then twist your hair around the base of the ponytail and clip it in place until it looks like a bun.

You may also braid your hair and tie only the end with a hair band.

Never use elastic bands with metal connectors or rubber bands on your hair. Always use soft material bands or soft grip clips. The less pressure on your hair the better.

When Bunning, don't tie the hair too tightly to minimize pressure on the hair.

While you are sleeping

Bunning or braiding can also be used as protective styles when you are sleeping. It's important to protect your hair as much as you can as tossing and turning causes friction which results in breakage, frizz and damage.

If you are comfortable with sleeping with something on your head, then wearing a satin scarf or hair net will also help.

If you, like myself can't bear to have anything on your head while you are sleeping and prefer to sleep with it loose, then invest in a satin pillowcase. This is one of the biggest luxuries a woman can indulge in. Not only does it keep your hair smooth while you sleep, it also protects the skin on your face. With no friction as you sleep, your skin is smooth without those morning wrinkles and lines that come from squashing your face while you sleep.

To preserve curly hair, make a very high ponytail and tie with a material covered hair scrunchie.

Refreshing natural dried hair

When you wake up, no matter how protected your hair, you might have to refresh the style.

The simplest way to do this is to wet your hands with water an a little conditioner or oil and smooth it over your hair shaft. Follow this up with either conditioner or light hair oil. This will instantly refresh the style and you are good to go without using heat.

If you have used heat and need to refresh the style, do not use the blow dryer again; rather wrap your hair with cling wrap as before. The best way to get the flat iron effect without the flat iron is to apply a good hair serum any one will do, and then brush your hair around your head as before. Apply the cling wrap or a stocking. Sit under a dryer for 15 minutes on medium heat. Then gently comb your hair out. Your hair will be extremely soft and have the straightened look without all the damage of a flat iron.

While you are exercising/sweating

It is important to tie hair up either in a high ponytail or hair bun whilst exercising. Wear a sweatband if you can stand it to absorb the moisture from your head. It is important to refresh the hair after exercising by combing it through with a wide toothcomb if your hair is straight or wavy, or with wet hand and a little conditioner if your hair is curly.

Don't touch your hair immediately after, allow the sweat to dry before manipulating hair so that it does not spread down the shaft of your hair.

While you are in the sun

Always wear a protective hat if you are outside in the sun. This is not only important for your skin but for your hair as well. It protects the hair from drying out.

If you are going swimming and do not want to wear a swimming cap, then ensure that you slather your hair with a rich leave in conditioner and apply more after swimming.
It's important to follow a wash routine following swimming. If you have a choice, choose to swim in a salt pool versus a chlorinated pool.

With heat

When you are trying to grow your hair, it is advisable to use heat as sparingly as possible. If you have to heat style your hair, then rather air dry first.

The best way to air dry hair if you plan to style it with heat, is to comb your hair around your head, this is called wrapping, and then putting a stocking or cling wrap over your hair. Allow to air dry to as dry as possible before using heat.

Some people's hair unfortunately cannot straighten from low or no heat settings, so if you must use heat, wait until your hair is as naturally dried as possible to minimize the amount of heat used on the hair.

Using curling or hot irons is never recommended. However if you must use a styling iron, do so only once a week and only on dry hair with a heat protection serum. Do not use styling irons if you have hair oil or silicone on your hair. You are literally frying your hair. The silicone will mask the damage until your next wash.

The best time to style your hair with heat, is after a moisturizing treatment when your hair is amply protected.

Without heat for curly or wavy hair

No heat is always the best option if you can get away with it. Some options to style your hair with no heat are the following:

- Plopping - for curly or wavy textures
- Apply a leave in conditioner, hair serum or light hair oil such as Coconut, Jojoba, Olive oil or Almond oil to your hair. You can also mix in a drop of pure honey for additional softness and shine.
- Comb through with a wide toothcomb or preferably your fingers.
- Spread an old t-shirt or micro-fiber towel onto a flat surface (such as the toilet with seat down).
- Bend over at the waist and position your hair in the middle of the cloth.
- Pile your hair to the top of your hair.
- With your head touching the cloth, drape the back section of cloth over your head.
- Twist the sides until they form "sausage rolls" and clip or tie them at the base of your neck.
- After 15-30 minutes remove the cloth. If your hair is frizzy after plopping lightly graze the hair with gel.
- Then remove the T shirt and shake your head gently
- Your hair will now have beautiful waves or curls depending on the texture of your hair
- After this - do not touch your hair at all. Any hair manipulation will cause your hair to frizz

Bunning or braiding - for any hair texture

Bunning is an easy style where you tie your hair up into a low or high ponytail, and then twist your hair around the base of the ponytail and clip it in place until it looks like a bun.

You may also braid your hair and tie only the end with a hair band.

Never use elastic bands with metal connectors or rubber bands on your hair. Always use soft material bands or soft grip clips. The less pressure on your hair the better.

When Bunning, don't tie the hair too tightly to minimize pressure on the hair.

While you are sleeping

Bunning or braiding can also be used as protective styles when you are sleeping. It's important to protect your hair as much as you can as tossing and turning causes friction which results in breakage, frizz and damage.

If you are comfortable with sleeping with something on your head, then wearing a satin scarf or hair net will also help.

If you, like myself can't bear to have anything on your head while you are sleeping and prefer to sleep with it loose, then invest in a satin pillowcase. This is one of the biggest luxuries a woman can indulge in. Not only does it keep your hair smooth while you sleep, it also protects the skin on your face. With no friction as you sleep, your skin is smooth without those morning wrinkles and lines that come from squashing your face while you sleep.

To preserve curly hair, make a very high ponytail and tie with a material covered hair scrunchie.

Refreshing natural dried hair

When you wake up, no matter how protected your hair, you might have to refresh the style.

The simplest way to do this is to wet your hands with water an a little conditioner or oil and smooth it over your hair shaft. Follow this up with either conditioner or light hair oil. This will instantly refresh the style and you are good to go without using heat.

If you have used heat and need to refresh the style, do not use the blow dryer again; rather wrap your hair with cling wrap as before. The best way to get the flat iron effect without the flat iron is to apply a good hair serum any one will do, and then brush your hair around your head as before. Apply the cling wrap or a stocking. Sit under a dryer for 15 minutes on medium heat. Then gently comb your hair out. Your hair will be extremely soft and have the straightened look without all the damage of a flat iron.

While you are exercising/sweating

It is important to tie hair up either in a high ponytail or hair bun whilst exercising. Wear a sweatband if you can stand it to absorb the moisture from your head. It is important to refresh the hair after exercising by combing it through with a wide toothcomb if your hair is straight or wavy, or with wet hand and a little conditioner if your hair is curly.

Don't touch your hair immediately after, allow the sweat to dry before manipulating hair so that it does not spread down the shaft of your hair.

While you are in the sun

Always wear a protective hat if you are outside in the sun. This is not only important for your skin but for your hair as well. It protects the hair from drying out.

If you are going swimming and do not want to wear a swimming cap, then ensure that you slather your hair with a rich leave in conditioner and apply more after swimming.
It's important to follow a wash routine following swimming. If you have a choice, choose to swim in a salt pool versus a chlorinated pool.

EMERGENCY HAIR RESCUE

When hair is severely damaged, the easy way out is to head straight for a big chop. This might the common answer but wait. Before cutting, follow this emergency hair regime:

For at least 2 months follow this regime religiously.

Emergency Treatment

1. First mix a 1/4 part honey, 1/4 part Extra Virgin Olive Oil and 1/2 any conditioner (as much as your hair needs)
2. Heat in the microwave for 10 seconds and stir.
3. Massage heated mixture into your dry or washed hair and leave in for 30 minutes to as long as you can stand it. Overnight is best.
4. Wash your hair with a gentle moisturizing sulfate free shampoo or conditioner.
Rinse out the treatment completely until the water runs clear.
Mix 2 teaspoons of Apple Cider Vinegar or Lemon juice to 2 cups of water and saturate your hair.
Blot your hair dry with a paper towel or micro fiber towel.
10. Apply a leave in treatment or conditioner. You may include a drop of honey into your leave in for extra shine and softness.
11. Comb through with a wide toothed comb or your fingers and air-dry your hair. Do not use any heat on your hair for as long as you can.
12. Sleep on a satin pillow case or cover your head with a satin scarf at night.

Hair and power nutrients

Our modern diets unfortunately do not provide all the nutrients Necessary not just for optimal, health but also for hair growth. Taking supplements in the form of vitamins is thus an essential part to achieve hair growth.

Based on scientific studies, there are a number of nutritional factors that can provide nutrients for beautiful and shiny hair and to sustain new hair growth. To really nourish and sustain healthy Hair growth, we must provide an internal Treatment, which contains high levels of the following active ingredients:

Sulphurated amino acids.

The two most critical sulphurated amino acids for new hair growth are L-methionine and L-cysteine which are essential building blocks for the formation of keratin (the basic structure of hair) and to promote hair growth.

B Vitamins

The B vitamins contribute to healthy skin and hair. B6 plays an important role in the absorption of the sulphurated aminoacids. Along with the B vitamins, vitamin E is an essential antioxidant associated both
Directly and indirectly in new hair growth.

Polyunsaturated fatty acids

The supercritical (CO2) millet seed (Panicum miliaceum) oil extract contains valuable linoleic acid, the triterpenoid miliacin as well as other phytosterols and squalene are important for sustaining hair growth. Clinical studies have proven it supports hair growth, has anabolic activity which supports the formation of lustrous and healthy hair.

Sunflower seed oil also contains valuable essential fatty acids of the omega 6 group that are necessary for the health of the hair. Sunflower seed oil can retain moisture in the skin and hair. It may also provide a protective barrier.

Silica

A lack of silica can lead to skin, nail and hair disorders as well as growth problems. A well-balanced hair formula should contain a good level of silica from horsetail. Additional silica can also prove to be extremely beneficial for the quality of hair and new hair growth. It can be used alongside other hair growth supplements.

Good Hair growth vitamins:

Vitamin A (as retinyl palmitate) 4000 IU
Vitamin E (natural mixed tocopherols) 45 IU
Riboflavin (Vitamin B2) 4 mg
Vitamin B6
Folic Acid 400 mcg (typically found in prenatal vitamins)
Biotin 1000 mcg,
Zinc (gluconate) 10 mg
L-Cysteine 100 mg,
L-Methionine 100 mg
Millet Seed Oil >6 mg of miliacin.

HEAD MASSAGE

Stimulating your hair follicles and blood vessels on your scalp is essential to stimulate hair growth. This is achieved in your prewash regime of massaging the head with oils.

You should however also massage your head daily for at least 5 minutes to deliver nutrients and oxygen to the hair follicles.

How to massage:

Push your scalp with your fingers in a circular motion as if washing; focus on each area for 30 seconds using both hands.
Choosing to go natural or not is a personal choice and no one should be condemned for that choice. It would be difficult to draw the line, as the word "natural" is open to interpretation. If my hair is naturally curly and I choose to flat iron or blow dry it once a month to straighten is, does this mean that I am no longer "natural". I personally choose both, at times I want to go all-natural, but if there's an occasion and I wish to wear a straight style, it is my choice.

My only advice on whether you choose to go natural or not, is that you always manage all risks of anything you do that goes against your natural texture or color that might damage your hair. This goes for blow drying, flat ironing, dyeing, hi-lighting, relaxing, perming etc.

THE TRUTH ABOUT RELAXERS

Relaxing

Any chemical process is damaging on your hair, however if you choose to go this route, then ensure that it is done on healthy hair. Relaxing over damaged, previously processed or bleached hair will cause your hair to break off or even disintegrate.

It is thus advisable that you first focus on treating your hair for as long as you can to get it into optimal health before relaxing.

Do not relax your hair more than once a month. Try to stretch out your relaxer to as long as possible as you focus on your hair regime and new growth. Always choose a mild relaxer.

The FDA in the United States lists Hair Dyes and Hair Strengtheners as the two top consumer complaints received in any given year! DIY Chemical processing products are available over any counter for anyone to use. It is however a powerful process which changes the basic chemical makeup of the hair strand.

Before performing any chemical process whether it's at home or in a salon, it is important to have all the information required to make informed decisions. The following information is scary - so be warned, natural doesn't sound that bad after reading this.

The History of Hair Strengtheners

Relaxers as we know it was accidentally discovered by Garrett Augustus Morgan, the son of former slaves. Hr also invented the traffic signal and gas mask! In 1910 while working in a sewing machine repair store attempting to invent a new lubricating liquid for the machine needle, legend has it that Morgan wiped his hands on a wool cloth, returned the next day, found the woolly texture of the cloth had smoothed out, and set out to find how the liquid chemical had changed the texture as it had. He experimented on an Airedale dog, known for their curly textured hair, and the effect was successfully duplicated.

Morgan then tried his lubricating liquid invention on himself, called it a "hair refining cream", and thus patented the first chemical hair straightener. He founded a personal grooming products company which included hair dying ointments, curved-tooth pressing combs, shampoo, hair pressing gloss, and the one that started it all: the "G.A. Morgan's Hair Refiner Cream" (advertised to "Positively Straighten Hair in 15 Minutes").

The truth behind Lye vs. No-Lye

Sodium Hydroxide is the strongest type of principal chemical used in some chemical relaxers because it provides the most long lasting and dramatic effects. However, this same sodium hydroxide is found in drain cleaners, which well demonstrate the strength of this, chemical. It is what is used in products that are referred to as "lye" relaxers. The strength varies from a pH factor of 10 to 14. With higher pH, the faster the straightening solution will take hold, but the more potential the damage.

Guanidine Hydroxide is the other common option of relaxer chemical used today. This is what is referred to as "no-lye" relaxers. This label can be misleading to some consumers. It does not imply that there aren't any strong chemicals used or that the chemicals used are somehow less potentially damaging. Some have mistakenly thought that with "no-lye" relaxers there are less steps and all the worry of chemical hair straightening is removed. Although this type of chemical hair relaxer can be less damaging than its counterpart, the hair and scalp should be in top condition before attempting treatment, and this type also requires special care when applied.

All relaxers require conditioning treatments before and after application. The decision to straighten the hair chemically requires much forethought and really a commitment to healthy hair care treatments over a long entire period of time.

The Do's / The Don'ts Before Relaxing

How can chemicals "relax", or straighten hair? Well first of all, as assumed, the chemical would need to be potent enough to do so. Both lye and "no lye" relaxers are very strong chemicals that work in the same manner by changing the basic structure of the hair shaft. The chemical penetrates the cortex and loosens the natural curl pattern. This inner layer of the hair shaft is not only what gives curly hair its shape but provides strength and elasticity. Once this process is performed it is irreversible.

This process which produces the desired effect of "straighter" hair at the same time leaves hair weak and extremely susceptible to breaking and further damage. One must keep in mind that relaxers do not help the hair, but actually strip it. So by applying chemicals to the hair, even if it is to achieve a desired effect, is never really to the benefit of your hair health.

Due to this, it is first strongly recommended that it be applied only under the direction of a hair care professional with a record of success with healthy hair care and chemical straightening, and that you follow conditioning treatments before and after the process.

Possessing a healthy scalp beforehand decreases the possibility of problems occurring. Relaxers should never be applied to already damaged hair, or on someone who has had scalp damage. Age should also be considered. Although your young children may want to have the hairstyles they see on adults or other young people, parents should seriously consider applying such strong chemicals to young hair and the potential damage that could last a lifetime if misused; most times it is not necessary to apply any chemical product to young hair.

"Over processing", the excessive use of relaxers on the hair or applying the chemical to already processed or relaxed hair, is the most typical misuse of these chemicals. Once the initial relaxer is applied to "virgin hair" (or a "virgin relaxer" is performed), "touch-ups" (or chemical applied thereafter) should only be applied to new growth between 6-8 week periods (or more). This however, depends on the rate of hair growth and condition of the hair as advised by your hair care professional. (Some say that even six weeks is too soon to reapply relaxer to new growth). And it is standard to wait at least 2-4 weeks before applying hair color chemical (or dye) to recently relaxed hair, if applied at all.

I've Decided to Straighten My Hair: Now What?

So after careful consideration you've decided to chemically straighten your hair. A "strand test" should always be performed during your consultation at the salon or on your own. Remember not all hair types (even if they are naturally tightly curled) are the same. Everyone's hair is different.

Tips when Relaxing Hair

Protective petroleum "base cream" should always be applied to help protect the scalp so that no chemical product comes in contact with your scalp. It should also be applied around the hairline and behind the ears.

After the relaxer chemical has been applied, and let set for the appropriate amount of time, the chemical needs to be completely removed with warm water, and then a neutralizing formula is applied. This step is essential to lower the pH – If not lowered the hair will break.

Apply a conditioner to restore some of the natural oils and proteins removed by the chemical.

Relaxers should be applied to hair that is completely dry.

Relaxers should be applied to unrelaxed hair only. Applying relaxer chemical to already relaxed hair will only cause breakage.

Do not exceed the processing time. It is crucial that this time period not be elapsed, as this will result in over-processing.

Scalp burning is not "normal", and when applied correctly the scalp should not burn. If you scalp burns, stop immediately.

If newly chemically straightened hair is not given special treatment it can become brittle, dry, damaged and break. Relaxed hair will tend to be drier and break easily. Regular deep conditioning is a must.

Limit the use of hot styling tools (such as blow dryers, hot combs, and curling irons). Try not to use heat on your hair at all between visits if possible.

Follow up a relaxer with a protein and moisture treatment.

Although there may be risks, and certainly much information to consider, in the hands of a professional, many have enjoyed for years good hair health while chemically straightening their hair. When done correctly this method does successfully straighten, soften the texture of the hair, and provides stunning results.

SUPER SECRETS FOR HAIR GROWTH

Amongst the various tips and tricks to maintaining healthy hair leading to growth - we all need that little extra secret that makes people go "Wow your hair has grown so quickly"! And here it is, the top secrets to super charge your hair growth.

Choose one or all and stick to it for at last one month. It's important to use one at a time so you can measure which one gives you faster growth. The hair treatments are all done as part of your bi-weekly wash routine but for emergency regrowth, e.g. after a bad hair cut or hair disaster - they can be done daily for the first week followed by twice a week thereafter.

Secret #1 - Vaginal Cream!

Many people that frequent hair forums have probably come across this at some point or another - however if you are new to growing your hair - then get ready for the long hair secret to faster growth that has worked on 90% on those that have tried it.

The secret is using Miconazole Nitrate - also known as Monistat or Daktarin in some countries - it is a vaginal anti-fungal cream!

In most well reported and documented cases, the hair on your head can indeed grow faster after using over the counter fungal cream. The key ingredient in these fungal creams used to treat vaginal yeast infections such as thrush or athletes foots, is Miconazole Nitrate (MN). An interesting side effect of MN is a boost in hair growth.

When I first read about this on a hair forum, I was intrigued by the sheer number of women who were raving about receiving growth of more than an inch within 1-2 weeks after massaging MN active creams into their scalps. After some research, I found that the ingredients used in these creams were also present in creams used to treat infant oral thrush.

The only side effect experienced by one in twenty women was mild to severe headaches. This was more prevalent in women who used undiluted 4% MN creams as opposed to women who diluted the cream with water. Most women who used a 2% solution did not report side effects.

Hair on average grows only half an inch per month on a healthy head of hair. For women to achieve 1-2 inches of growth is decidedly above average.

Curious to test this interesting theory, I purchased two boxes of Daktarin Vaginal Cream at my local pharmacy. Granted, I felt slight discomfort when asking for two boxes, while the lady at the counters face evidently questioned why I needed two boxes when one should suffice. I was ready to justify my purchase, but unfortunately did not need to.

I started on January 9th with plans to use the cream 1-3 times a week for one month. Ladies on the hair forums alternated between using it once a week to every night. Results between the groups were negligible, so I took the mean, one to three times a week.

I measured my head from the mid-front of my hairline, to the longest point of my hair at the back. I measured several times using a normal tape measure, to ensure that my measurements would be accurate. My hair measured at 20".

You apply a small amount of the Monistat/Daktarin cream onto fingertips, tip your head over and massaged it into your scalp. Repeat until entire scalp is massaged.

For the first week, there was no noticeable growth. In the second week, my hair somehow felt longer and thicker. I put this down to the placebo effect. Strangely though, I was struggling to see through my fringe. My fringe was slightly past eyebrow level; suddenly it was brushing against the bridge of my nose.
As the weeks until the 9th February dragged on, I continued my normal hair routines, but applied the MN religiously one to three times a week dependent on my mood. I also mixed it with Castor Oil in the middle of my trial period as someone had reported easier application.

Barely 3 weeks into my trial, 7 days shy of 9 February, I decided to cheat and measure my hair. At this point it was no longer my imagination, my hair was longer.
Upon measuring the same distance, from my hairline to the longest point of my hair at the back, my hair now measured 21". I re-measured several times again to ensure an accurate result.

In 3 weeks my hair had grown an inch. I also normally massage my head with oils, including castor oil, so the growth could not be attributed to this alone.

Based on results of others and more importantly my own trial, I can say that, YES, a vaginal fungal cream can make your hair grow faster.

Secret #2 - Emu Oil Hair Growth

The following recipe has proven to speed up hair growth. Personally it's a bit thick for me, but many women have found that it works.

Ingredients
3 Tablespoons Emu Oil
5 Tablespoons Extra Virgin Olive Oil
5 Tablespoons Castor Oil
5 Tablespoons Raw Honey

Mix all ingredients together in a blender for 2 minutes on medium high speed, or better yet, use one of those hand held blenders. After you've mixed everything together, place in a clean glass container with an airtight lid. I use a small mason jar. Keep refrigerated!

Grease your scalp with this mixture for 7 days straight. At the end of 7 days you can wash your hair. VERY IMPORTANT ~ you MUST massage your scalp once per day for at least 3-5 minutes. This will help the oils penetrate the scalp. If you skip this important step in the treatment process, you might not see the best results.

Secret #3 - Grow Hair Like A Weed Oil!

This recipe is probably one of the best oil mixtures to speed up hair growth. Due to the thickness of the mixture, the regime is not easy to incorporate into daily life, however if you need to re-grow after a hair emergency then this will give you a head start. Your hair will double in growth rate.

Ingredients for one weeks worth
1/4-Cup Extra Virgin Olive Oil
1/4-Cup Pure Coconut Oil
1/4 Cup Almond Oil
1/4 Cup Avocado Oil
1/4 Cup Amla Indian Hair Oil (optional)

1 Teaspoon of melted Honey

Mix all ingredients together and pour into a jar or bottle. Massage the mixture into your hair 3-4 times a week. Continue to follow your hair regime as normal, using this as your pre-oiling. The only difference is that you have to leave these oils on your head and only wash on your washdays. Use an Apple Cider Vinegar rinse to clarify the hair.

The oils can be bought at an Organic store, Whole Foods, Dischem or BJs depending o your area. Any health store will stock the oils in its purest forms.
This mixture is probably one of the best options in conjunction with the Monistat/Daktarin to really speed up hair growth. It also super conditions your hair, makes it shiny, fortified, reconstructed, moisturized, softened and de-frizzed.

You can also add Rosemary essential oil (about 20 drops) and MSM powder.

HOME MADE RECIPES

The following is a list of natural hair and personal care recipes. The recipes can be tweaked according to what works for your hair. Try them with your hair routine to see what works for you.

Warning: Do not use heat when using deep conditioner treatments with raw egg. Simply cover the hair and leave on without heat!

Shampoo

Chamomile Shampoo

4 Bags of chamomile tea
4 tablespoons of soap flakes (available at beauty stores or drug stores)
1 1/2 tablespoon of glycerin.

Steep the 4 bags of tea in 1 1/2 cups of boiling water. Remove the tea bags and with the remaining liquid add the soap flakes. Let stand until the soap softens. Stir in glycerin until mixture is well blended. Pour into a bottle. Keep in a dark, cool place.

Dry Shampoo

If you need to refresh oily hair but do not have time to wash or are extending your washdays - then the best home dry shampoo is simple cornstarch. Simple sprinkle some into your scalp and hair then brush out. The cornstarch will absorb excess oil.

Simple Shampoo

1/4-cup water
1/4-cup liquid Castile Soap
1/2-teaspoon sunflower or other light vegetable oil

Mix together all the ingredients. Store in a bottle. Use as you would any shampoo, rinse well.
Beer Shampoo
3/4-cup beer (any brand)
1-cup inexpensive shampoo

Boil the beer until it reduces to 1/4 cup. Cool the beer and add it to the 1-cup of inexpensive shampoo. Shampoo hair as normal.

Conditioners

Tropical Conditioner

1 peeled and mashed Avocado
1 cup Coconut milk

Combine mashed avocado with some coconut milk in a small bowl. Heat in microwave for approx. 45 seconds. Stir. Test temperature. Massage mixture into hair. Wrap hair in a hot towel or cover with shower cap for 15 minutes. Shampoo & rinse out.

Jojoba Hair Conditioner

1 cup rose floral water
1-tablespoon jojoba oil
10 drops vitamin E oil

In the top of a double boiler, gently warm the rose water. Once rose water is warm, add jojoba oil. For extra conditioning, leave on for several minutes. Rinse thoroughly with warm water. Shampoo and rinse again with cool water.

Honey Conditioner

2 Tbsps olive oil
1 tsp honey
1 egg yolk.
Mix all ingredients in small bowl. Massage on hair in small sections. Wrap head with shower cap for 30 minutes. Rinse and shampoo.

Egg Conditioner

1 egg yolk
1/2 tsp olive oil
3/4-cup lukewarm water

Beat egg yolk until it is thick and light colored. Add oil beat well. Slowly add and beat the water into the egg mixture. Pour mixture into a container. After shampooing, massage all conditioner into hair and leave on for a few minutes before thoroughly rinsing.

Mayonnaise Conditioner

1/2-cup mayo

Rinse and towel dry. Apply mayonnaise to the hair. Massage in. Let sit for 10-15 minutes, shampoo again lightly and rinse with an apple cider vinegar and water solution. This will help with the smell and remove any residue.

Sesame & Coconut Protein Conditioner

2 tbsp olive oil
2 tbsp light sesame oil
2 eggs
2 tbsp coconut milk
2 tbsp honey
1 tsp coconut oil

Mix ingredients in bowl, apply to hair before shampoo. Let sit for 20 minutes. Rinse, then shampoo.

Avocado Conditioner

1 small jar of mayonnaise
1/2 avocado

Peel avocado and remove pit. Mash avocado then mix all ingredients in a medium-sized bowl with your hands until it's a consistent green color. Smooth into hair. Use shower cap or plastic wrap to seal body heat in. Leave on hair for 20 minutes. For deeper conditioning wrap a hot, damp towel around your head over the plastic, or use a hair dryer set to a low to medium heat setting. Store extra in refrigerator.

Olive oil conditioner

1/2-cup olive oil
1/2 cup boiling water
Combine ingredients then warm on low heat. Massage mixture into the scalp and hair. Wrap hair in a hot towel for 15 minutes. Shampoo & rinse out.

Banana Conditioner

1/2 a banana
1/4 avocado
1/4 cantaloupe
1-tablespoon wheat germ oil
1-tablespoon yogurt

Blend all ingredients. Apply to hair. For extra conditioning, squeeze in the contents of a vitamin E capsule. Leave in hair for 15 minutes. Then rinse.

Coconut Oil Conditioner

4 tbls Coconut Oil
2 tbls Natural honey

Place coconut oil and honey in a small plastic bag and place the bag in a hot cup of water for 1 minute to warm. Apply to hair; wrap hair in a towel for 20 minutes. Wash then dry hair.

Coconut Honey Deep Conditioner

1-tablespoon virgin olive oil
2 tablespoons honey
1-tablespoon buttermilk
1-tablespoon natural unbleached flour

Blend all ingredients. Microwave the mixture for 30 seconds until hot. Stir in one tablespoon of natural unbleached flour to make a paste. Apply the warm paste to wet hair and allow the conditioner to set for 20 minutes Wash as normal.

Strength Building Deep Conditioner

1-teaspoon honey
4 cups (1 quart) warm water
Squeeze of lemon juice

Mix ingredients. After shampooing, pour mixture through hair. Do not rinse out. Dry as normal.

Chamomile Conditioner

6 chamomile tea bags
1/2-cup plain yogurt
Lavender oil
Bring one cup of water to boil and steep tea bags for 15 minutes. Discard tea bags. Combine yogurt and 7 drops of lavender oil with chamomile tea, mix thoroughly. Apply the mixture to dry hair, working through to ends. Cover head in plastic wrap and condition for thirty minutes. Shampoo hair.

Color Enhancers

Blonde Highlights

1 cup lemon juice
3 cups chamomile tea (brewed, & cooled)

Mix ingredients, pour over damp hair then let sit for an hour while you sit in the sun, wash out. Follow with a good conditioner. Do this a few times a week to notice the highlights.

Brunettes- Black coffee or tea

Brew coffee or tea. Allow to cool. Pour overhead. Let set or 15 min. Then apply again. Rinse well.

Red Heads

1/2-cup beet juice
1/2-cup carrot juice

Mix ingredients together, pour over clean, damp hair. Wrap head in plastic and apply hot towel, medium dryer heat, or sit in the sun for one hour. Shampoo then condition.

Henna Color

Henna color in powder form
Your Favorite Deep conditioner

Mix henna using half the water as directed on the package. Add your favorite deep conditioner to the mixture. Apply to hair, working through hair thoroughly. Leave on hair following directions as indicated on package. Shampoo. May be used with colorless henna to increase volume of fine hair without adding color.

To Darken Brunettes

1/3 cup walnut shells, black tea, cherry tree bark or cloves
2 1/2 cups water

Add ingredients to a non-metal bowl or pot. Use a double broiler for this. Simmer ingredients in water 20 minutes. Remove from heat, strain ingredients, saving liquid in an old shampoo bottle. Apply to hair as a final rinse.
Herbs for conditioning and highlighting LIGHT hair
Marigold flowers, chamomile flowers, nettle, rhubarb root, safflower, mullein flowers
Herbs for conditioning and accentuating DARK hair
Bay leaves, black walnut hulls, burdock root, nettle, quassia bark, cloves, cinnamon

Natural Honey Lightening

2 Tbsp Honey (Raw dark colored honey works best)
6 Tbsp Distilled Water

Mix the honey and water and let it sit for one hour out of sunlight or use immediately.
Use on wet or dry freshly washed hair with no leave in product on the hair.
Apply the mixture to hair with a dye brush or spray bottle.
The wet must remain completely wet - once applied cover with cling wrap (saran wrap) or a swim cap to keep the hair wet. Do not use a towel or any other item that will absorb the water.
Leave on the hair for 1 hour and rinse.

If hair is crunchy - follow up with an Apple Cider Vinegar rinse. This is as a result of honey residue on the hair. The honey has natural peroxide, which will be released into your hair, without the damage. It is also a great conditioner and humectants (attracts moisture) for your hair.
The longer you do this, the lighter your hair will become. Thus you can do this every day if you want to. This is not a drastic method, your hair won't suddenly be blonde - but it will create natural highlights in your hair that is 1-2 shades lighter than your natural color.

Scalp Treatments

Brown Sugar Head Scrub

If you have dandruff, flakes or even an oily scalp, this scrub will remove all impurities.
4 tbls of Brown Sugar
2 tbls of your favorite conditioner

Combine brown sugar and conditioner in a bowl and mix well. Apply to scalp only with fingers! Scrub scalp in a circular motion for a few minutes. Rinse, then shampoo and condition as normal.

Deep Conditioner Treatments

Super Deep Hot Oil Conditioner Recipe
1 tablespoons Avocado Oil
2 tablespoons Coconut Oil
8 drops Chamomile Roman Essential oil
8 drops Myrrh Essential oil

Place oils in a small plastic bag and place the bag in a hot cup of water for 1 minute to warm. Apply to hair; wrap hair in a towel for 20 minutes. Wash then dry hair.

Silky, Shiny Hot Oil Hair Recipe

1 tablespoon Coconut oil
1 tablespoon Almond oil
1 teaspoon Evening primrose oil
1 tablespoon Jojoba oil
5 drops Rosemary Essential oil
5 drops Chamomile Roman Essential oil

Melt coconut oil if not liquid. Add other carrier oils, allow to cool then add Essential Oils. Apply to hair; wrap hair in a towel for 30-45 minutes. Wash then dry hair.

Avocado Deep Condition

1 small jar of mayonnaise
1/2 avocado

Peel avocado and remove pit. Mash avocado then mix all ingredients in a medium-sized bowl with your hands until it's a consistent green color. Smooth into hair. Use shower cap or plastic wrap to seal body heat in. Leave on hair for 20 minutes. For deeper conditioning wrap a hot, damp towel around your head over the plastic, or use a hair dryer set to a low to medium heat setting. Store extra in refrigerator.

Hot Oil Deep Treatment

1/2-cup olive oil
1/2 cup boiling water
Combine ingredients then warm on low heat. Massage mixture into the scalp and hair. Wrap hair in a hot towel for 15 minutes. Shampoo & rinse out.

Fruity Deep Conditioner

1/2 a banana
1/4 avocado
1/4 cantaloupe
1-tablespoon wheat germ oil
1-tablespoon yogurt
Blend all ingredients. Apply to hair. For extra conditioning, squeeze in the contents of a vitamin E capsule. Leave in hair for 15 minutes. Then rinse.

Strength Building Deep Conditioner

1-tablespoon virgin olive oil
2 tablespoons honey
1-tablespoon buttermilk
1-tablespoon natural unbleached flour

Blend all ingredients. Microwave the mixture for 30 seconds until hot. Stir in one tablespoon of natural unbleached flour to make a paste. Apply the warm paste to wet hair and allow the conditioner to set for 20 minutes Wash as normal.

Honey & Olive Oil

1-tablespoon honey
1 tablespoon Extra Virgin Olive oil
2 tablespoons of any conditioner

You can double up these quantities for longer hair. Stir the mixture with a plastic spoon. Heat in the microwave for 10 seconds or over a cup of hot water until the mixture congeals into a paste. Apply to your hair. Cover your hair with a shower cap or hot towel. Leave on for minimum 30-60 minutes.

Henna

Natural henna is a great conditioner, thickener and color enhancer. Mix 1 packet natural skin grade henna with water and olive oil to form a paste. Apply to hair and leave on for 1 hour. Rinse, wash and condition as usual. As natural henna is drying, it is best to apply it with the olive oil to counteract the drying effect.

Increased hair growth conditioning treatment

Mix a vial of bergamot essence (available at pharmacies) with a bottle of bay rum about 100ml (medicinal available at pharmacies) into a spray bottle. Spray the mixture as a leave in into your hair as often as possible. Alternatively throw a vial of the bergamot essence into your regular conditioner.

Hair Growth Hot Oil Treatment Recipe

2 oz jojoba oil
5 drops of essential oil of Sage
8 drops of essential oil of Rosemary

Place oils in a small plastic bag and place the bag in a hot cup of water for 1 minute to warm. Apply to hair; wrap hair in a towel for 20 minutes. Wash then dry hair.

Rosemary Hot Oil Treatment

1/2 ounce Coconut oil
1/2 ounce Castor oil
1/2 ounce Emu oil
1/2 ounce Jojoba, natural
1/3 once Broccoli seed oil
1/2 ounce Arnica oil
15 drops Rosemary essential oil

Massage mixture into damp hair. Wrap hair in a hot towel or cover with shower cap for 20 minutes. Shampoo & rinse out.

Rosemary Almond Hot Oil Treatment

4 1/2 Oz. Almond Oil
4 Drops Rosemary Essential Oil
4 Drops Lavender Essential Oil

Massage mixture into damp hair. Wrap hair in a hot towel or cover with shower cap for 20 minutes. Shampoo & rinse out.

Hair Rinses

Apple Cider Vinegar Rinse

1/2 cup Apple Cider Vinegar
1 jug water

Mix the apple cider vinegar and water. Use as a final hair rinse after conditioning.

Apple Cider Vinegar removes build-up and residue from the hair shaft and closes the cuticles. Vinegar also prevents an itchy scalp. Although plain white vinegar works fine, apple cider vinegar works better. The smell goes away once your hair dries!

Apple Cider Softening Hair Rinse

Mix 1-2 tablespoons apple cider vinegar with 3 cups distilled water.

Pour over your hair as the final rinse after conditioning. It will leave your hair feeling soft.

Shiny Hair Rinse

Mix the juice from 1/2 lemon, 2 tablespoons of apple cider vinegar and 1 cup of water.

Shampoo and rinse hair as usual, then pour the mixture on your hair and massage into the scalp. Rinse with cool water.

Anti-Frizz For All Hair Types

1 tsp Fresh Lemon Juice
2 cups (500ml) Tap Water

Wash and conditioner your hair. Use the mixture as a rinse; be sure to saturate all hair with the mixture. Great anti-frizz cure and curl/wave definer.

Dandruff Remedies

The shedding of dead skin cells on the scalp causes dandruff - it is not dry scalp. Dandruff is caused by some of the following:
- Excessive exposure to extreme heat or cold
- Overuse of products such as gel or hairspray

- Ill health
- Constipation
- Stress
- Harsh Shampoos
- General exhaustion

In addition to the remedies below avoid citrus foods, bananas, coffee, tea, processed food, refined and tinned foods that aggravate dandruff.

The following remedies will assist with ridding your scalp of dandruff.

Dandruff Powder

Massage handfuls of baking soda into the hair and scalp to absorb oil and to loosen dead skin on scalp. Rinse thoroughly, use no other shampoos. While initially the hair may seem dry, after several weeks, dandruff will be gone and hair will be smooth and shiny.

Dandruff Mint Rinse

1-cup water
1-cup apple cider vinegar
1 handful of fresh mint leaves

Boil ingredients. Strain and pour into a container. Massage solution into the scalp, let dry without rinsing out

Dandruff Vinegar Rinse

One of the best ways to control dandruff is to apply a mixture of normal vinegar and water to the scalp.
Apply warm coconut oil on the scalp with a cotton ball as part of your pre-wash oiling routine. Leave it overnight. Apply the juice of a lemon on the scalp the next morning and wash your hair as usual after 30 minutes.

Stinky Dandruff Treatment!
Mix 1 part sulfur powder, 2 parts surgical spirits, 1 part almond oil
and 4 parts rose water, or distilled water. Rub on your scalp.

Olive Oil Dandruff Treatment

Mix some olive oil and almond oil and massage into your scalp.
Leave for 5 minutes then rinse.

TOP 5 HAIR GROWTH KILLERS

No matter how tempted you are - avoid the following as much as possible, these are the top 5 hair killers, with safer alternatives I've recommended. These are all from experience; trust me I've been here!

1. Going more than 3 shades lighter than your own hair color. This is a no no. There is only one way to get hair that light, no matter what they tell you, and that's bleach. They might call it peroxide or lighteners or toners or whatever - bottom line is that they are bleaching your hair. Bleaching takes color out of the hair, thus significantly thinning your hair strand making it more susceptible to breakage. If you must - then ensure that you get a deep protein treatment before and after to protect hair as much as possible. Even then your hair will still be weakened, so will take a lot of deep conditioning to maintain.
2. Hair extensions. As tempting as it might be to have instantly longer hair - most hair extensions whether it's a synthetic bond or metal bond - results in hair breaking off. The weight of the extension on your natural hair creates tension, which weakens the hair. If you must, then opt for a clip in and don't wear them too often. You can also opt for mini hairpieces or half wigs to add volume or body.
3. Dyeing your hair more than once in 6 weeks. Dye adds color to hair but also changes the chemical composition resulting

in dry hair. If you must, then ensure that you deep treat your hair before and after.

4. Chemical processing - i.e. relaxing, perming, keratin treatments, Brazilian blowout - no matter the name, the marketing or the hype - these are all chemical processes, and none of them are safe. They are all temporary processes that cause damage to your hair and health. Inhalation of these chemicals alone can lead to severe health effects. There is no such thing as a safe chemical process. If you must - then again ensure that your hair is at optimal health and that you are deep treating before and after. This is no guarantee that you will prevent damage; you will only be trying to fix the damage you know you are causing!

5. Major chops! Avoid going for major on impulse. Your hair condition can improve with micro trims and following a strict hair routing. If you get an impulse to chop your hair off - follow the next day rule. First wash and deep condition your hair followed by a micro trim, no more than 1/8" on dry hair. The next day you can decide whether you still want to cut it.

TOP 50 HAIR GROWTH RULES

1. Comb tangled hair with a wide tooth comb only
2. Do not brush wet hair
3. Do not use rubber bands or metal clips on the hair. Use only material covered bands
4. Air dry your hair as much as possible
5. Limit the use of heat appliances to as little as possible, once a week if you must
6. Wear hair up as much as possible to protect the ends (Bunning)
7. Minimize shampoo regimes to twice a week
8. Try to alternate by shampooing your hair with conditioner once a week
9. Avoid chemical processes as much as possible
10. Try to use boar bristle brushes which are gentler on hair
11. Do not use hot water when rinsing
12. Use cold water as your final rinse to seal the cuticles for a healthy shine
13. Add crushed garlic cloves to your conditioner to minimize hair shedding
14. Use Miconzole Nitrate products (normally used for vaginal yeast infections e.g. Monistat, Daktarin) and massage into your scalp as part of your prewashing regime to increase growth (more information further on)
15. Do not sleep on polyester or cotton pillowcases. Try to purchase a silk satin case and sleep on this
16. Alternatively purchase a satin scarf or head turban to cover your hair when sleeping/showering
17. Comb your hair with a wide tooth comb as soon as tangles are felt
18. Stretch out trims to 6 weeks and only trim 1/8" of the split ends nothing else

19. Do micro trims of split ends as soon as you notice them at least weekly
20. Drink a minimum of 8 glasses a water a day
21. Try to exercise for a minimum of 15-20 minutes three times a week
22. Sauna or any method of getting steam into the head contributes to hair growth
23. Doing a mini micro trim on the evening of a New Moon. This moon phase has proved to be beneficial to encourage hair growth
24. Apply leave in silicone, Jojoba, Coconut Oil or hair serum to the ends of hair every night
25. Use a micro fiber turban hair towel to dry hair
26. Do not rub hair vigorously after washing, rather twist your hair turban style into a towel or use a turban towel to soak up the excess water
27. Drink Green Tea daily
28. Eat foods rich in protein
29. Treat hair like silk
30. Try not to touch your hair too much
31. Do not use sprays or silicones when using heating appliances. Use a leave in heat protectant, and allow to air dry before using a blow-dryer or iron
32. Do not use hair spray which contains high concentration of alcohol which dries hair
33. Put shampoo on your fingertips and wash the scalp only with fingertips - then smooth hair with palm of hands. Focus on scalp when you wash, the lengths and ends will get clean from the soap suds that run down from your scalp.
34. Use only one dollop of shampoo, more is not required.
35. Use sulfate free hair products. Sulfates causes build up which causes frizz and crunchy ends.
36. The Zone diet has a side effect of faster hair growth, which can be attributed to the high protein side of the diet. Adding more protein into your diet is thus beneficial to faster and healthier hair growth.
37. Massage your scalp daily as this assists with the blood flow to your scalp.

38. Alcohol and smoking influences hair loss. Try to cut down or cut out both of these habits.
39. Stress is a major contributor to hair loss. Find things to do to help you de-stress such as exercise, yoga, meditation, praying, reading a book, watching a comedy - anything that takes your mind off worrying
40. Aloe Vera gel or liquid is a great frizz treatment and also aids with hair loss and promotes hair growth.
41. Adding rosemary essential oil to your conditioner will also promote hair growth as it stimulates the scalp.
42. When buying hair products, look for the following ingredients, which are beneficial to hair growth: Aloe Vera, Citrus Fruits, Jojoba, Rosemary and Sage.
43. Stay away from products that have "Extracts". They are not as powerful as essential oils, which are concentrated.
44. Never use hair accessories that have metal, whether it's a clip, slide, grip or spring. Use only soft plastic or material covered accessories, and opt for silky material coverings. Hair sticks are great but buy high quality ones with no joins that can tangle or break the hair.
45. Avoid chemical processes - embrace your natural texture and nurture it to look it's best.
46. Comb your hair BEFORE shampooing to remove knots.
47. If you have dry or curly hair, always use a leave in conditioner, serum or oil. It acts as a sealant, thus sealing in moisture.
48. Try to use more organic or homemade products.
49. Use deep protein treatments at least once a month followed by a high quality moisturizing treatment. A simple egg will do.
50. Avoid spraying perfume into your hair as the alcohol has a drying effect on the hair.

SAMPLE HAIR CARE ROUTINE

The next pages are your free sample hair routine/regime checklist and journal to keep track of your progress with space for photos and inspiration.

It also includes a list of daily routines you can do. Not all are necessary, but for optimal hair growth, try to do as many as you can.

It is important to stick to a routine - or try to for at least 2 months and you will see a difference!

My ideal washdays are Tuesdays and Saturdays; yours might differ but choose two days and try to stick to them.

It is recommended to print the routine and journal page (as many as you need) and keep them in one file.

This is a sample routine and can be adapted to suit your needs / lifestyle / preferences. The routine in the journal is blank to allow you to either copy the sample routine or make up your own. You can re-print it as your needs change

Hair Routine

Wash Day 1

- o Preoil your dry unwashed hair by massaging any hair oils (preferably pure Coconut Oil) into the scalp, lengths and ends of your hair
- o Cover with a wrap or hot towels for 30 minutes or under a dryer for 15 minutes.
- o Wash your hair once with a gentle sulphate free shampoo or conditioner if you do not want to use shampoo.
- o Apply a Moisturizing Conditioner/Treatment.
- o Comb through with a wide tooth comb
- o Cover your hair with a hot towel or shower cap and sit under a dryer for 15 minutes or leave covered for 30 minutes.
- o Rinse thoroughly with luke warm then cold water to seal the cuticles.
- o Seal in moisture by using a hair serum, leave in conditioner, Extra Virgin olive oil, coconut oil, amla indian oil, almond oil or avocado oil.
- o Style hair

Wash Day 2

- o Preoil your dry unwashed hair by massaging any hair oils (preferably pure Coconut Oil) into the scalp, lengths and ends of your hair
- o Cover with a wrap or hot towels for 30 minutes or under a dryer for 15 minutes.
- o Wash your hair once with a gentle sulphate free shampoo or conditioner if you do not want to use shampoo.

o Apply a Protein Conditioner/Treatment for 30 minutes and cover your hair. 15 minutes if you are using a dryer.
o Rinse and apply a Moisturizing Conditioner or Treatment
o Comb through with a wide tooth comb
o Cover your hair with a hot towel or shower cap and sit under a dryer for 15 minutes or leave covered for 30 minutes.
o Rinse thoroughly with luke warm then cold water to seal the cuticles.
o Seal in moisture by using a hair serum, leave in conditioner, Extra Virgin olive oil, coconut oil, amla Indian oil, almond oil or avocado oil.
o Style hair

Daily Regime

The daily regime should be followed every single day whether it's washday or not.

1. Take your own choice of vitamins for hair growth daily
2. Comb through and cover hair before sleeping or sleep on a silk pillowcase
3. Drink 8 glasses of water
4. Try to do some form of exercise for a minimum of 15 minutes or head stands for 5 minutes
5. Massage your head without oil for 5 minutes daily
Apply a serum or coconut oil to the ends daily

Optional to super charge hair growth.

You may apply the Secret hair growth mixtures Monistat, the Emu Oil or Grow Hair Like A Weed mixtures to your scalp 2-3 times a week in between washdays. The oiling and Monistat mixtures can be done together without adverse effects. Distribution of both mixtures are done best on wet hair, but can also be done on dry hair.

EMBRACE YOUR CURLZ

For curly hair types (normally from hair type 3a onwards) - hair needs special care. Due to the texture of the hair, curly hair is a lot more porous than straight hair and thus more prone to dryness and frizz.

All the hair care tips in this book still apply to curly hair, however the curly hair routine will take your curls to a different level! Before we get to the routine a few curly hair secrets to fabulous hair.

No Poo!

Curly hair does not respond well to sulphate shampoo, so this is the first thing that has to go. Sulphate laden shampoos dry out straight hair, so you can imagine what it does to holey curly hair. Sulfates are the same ingredient in dishwashing liquids and other household detergents! It's going to be very hard to do this, but for the sake of healthy hair, you will have to try. Instead you will now follow the CO washing method, which is to wash your hair with a light conditioner. If done properly, you will not feel as if your hair is heavy or unclean. The trick to washing your hair with conditioner (any light cheap conditioner) is to use conditioner the exact same way, as you would shampoo, however let the conditioner sit in your hair for longer before you rinse. You have to also rub the scalp a bit harder to loosen the dirt and grime, however it will come clean. You follow up with a deeper conditioner as you normally would an Apple Cider Vinegar or Lemon Juice rinse. This last step is important!

However before you start on your new Curly Hair routine - do a clarifying wash with shampoo as your first and only shampoo wash to rid your hair of any product build up.

It is important to note that it can take up to 6 weeks for your hair to settle into this new routine, although for most it's a lot quicker. Be patient - you will see results!

Silicones

When selecting conditioners to use on your curly hair, try to go for ones that have soluble silicones:

Silicones that are not soluble in water and build up on the hair (bad cones)
Cetearyl methicone, Cetyl Dimethicone, Cyclomethicone, Cyclopentasiloxane, Dimethicone, Dimethiconol, Stearyl Dimethicone, Amodimethicone (and) Trideceth-12 (and) Cetrimonium Chloride, and Trimethylsilylamodimethicone. Note: Trideceth-12 and Cetrimonium Chloride are only considered a silicone when both are combined with Amodimethicone.

Silicones that are slightly soluble in water and will build up on most types of curly hair
Amodimethicone, Behenoxy Dimethicone, and Stearoxy Dimethicone.

Silicones that is soluble in water and safe to use (they are not listed with PEG in front of them)

Dimethicone Copolyol, Hydrolyzed Wheat Protein Hydroxypropyl Polysiloxane, and Lauryl methicone copolyol. [10]

Silicones that have the letters "PEG" in front of them mean that the silicones are water soluble so will rinse out and not as damaging as non soluble silicones.

Curly Hair Routine

Wash Day 1

- o Preoil your dry unwashed hair by massaging any hair oils (the Grow Hair Like A Weed recipe works well here but do it the night before) into the scalp, lengths and ends of your hair. You can also do this on damp hair.
- o Cover with a wrap or hot towels for 30 minutes or under a dryer for 15 minutes or if you did this the night before and slept on it you can skip this step.
- o Wash your hair once with a gentle cheap conditioner. Let it sit on your hair and work through your scalp, mid lengths and ends.
- o Apply another Moisturizing Conditioner/Treatment.
- o Comb through with a wide tooth comb
- o Rinse thoroughly with luke warm.
- o Rinse with a teaspoon of Apple Cider Vinegar or Fresh Lemon Juice in 2 cups of water.
- o Apply conditioner or any styling product that you prefer as a leave in. Do not comb the hair vigorously, only gently manipulate and scrunch with your fingers into the style you desire.
- o Air-dry as much as possible - if you are in a hurry air-dry most of your hair and finish off with a diffuser to minimize damage.

Wash Day 2

- o Preoil your dry unwashed hair by massaging any hair oils (preferably pure Coconut Oil) into the scalp, lengths and ends of your hair
- o Cover with a wrap or hot towels for 30 minutes or under a dryer for 15 minutes.
- o Wash your hair once with a gentle conditioner.
- o Apply a Protein Conditioner/Treatment for 30 minutes and cover your hair. 15 minutes if you are using a dryer.
- o Rinse and apply a Moisturizing Conditioner or Treatment
- o Comb through with a wide tooth comb
- o Cover your hair with a hot towel or shower cap and sit under a dryer for 15 minutes or leave covered for 30 minutes.
- o Rinse thoroughly with luke warm then cold water to seal the cuticles.
- o Do a final rinse with a mixture of 1 teaspoon fresh squeezed lemon juice or Apple Cider Vinegar and 2 cups of water.
- o Air-dry as much as possible - if you are in a hurry air-dry most of your hair and finish off with a diffuser to minimize damage.
- o You may apply conditioner or leave in as required, however the lemon rinse will give your curls definition.
- o Style hair as usual using fingers, scrunching or plopping.

Daily Regime

The daily regime should be followed every single day whether it's washday or not.

1. Take your own choice of vitamins for hair growth daily
Before going to bed, spray hair until damp with water, apply coconut oil on the ends. Plop hair (see Styling section).
When you wake up refresh hair by spraying with a light mixture of water and conditioner or water and aloe Vera/jojoba oil.

Drink 8 glasses of water
4. Try to do some form of exercise for a minimum of 15 minutes or head stands for 5 minutes
5. Massage your head without oil for 5 minutes daily
Apply a serum or coconut oil to the ends daily

CONCLUSION

Good luck on your hair growth journey. Remember - whatever you focus on increases - so focus on having beautiful, long and healthy hair and be committed to your journey.